Paleo Diet

Simple Paleo Diet Recipes For Rapid Weight Loss

(Paleo Diet Recipes For Beginners)

Rick Sandoval

TABLE OF CONTENTS

Whip Gluten-Free Banana Pancakes 1

Prosciutto Wrapped Chicken 2

Green Paleo Smoothie 3

Beef Skewers And 8oz Of Water 4

Breakfast Paleo Waffles 7

Hungry Man Steak And Bacon Hash 9

No-Crust Mini Bacon Quiches 11

Pumpkin Breakfast Pancakes 13

Poblano Pepper Omelet 15

Jalapeño Scrambled Fresh Eggs With Cherry Tomatoes 16

Peachy Pancakes 19

Mexican Scramble 20

Healthy Granola Bars 22

Paleo Beef Jerky 24

Spicy Nuts 25

Veggie-Bun Sandwich 28

Low-Carb Paleo Patties And 8oz Of Water 29

Walnut Pesto Chicken Salad 31

Grilled Chicken Salad 32

Chicken And Broccoli Salad 34

Vitamin Chicken Salad 35

Chicken, Lettuce And Avocado Salad 36

Mashed Avocado And Chicken Salad 38

Easy Chicken And Egg Salad 39

Mediterranean Chicken Soup 40

Chicken And Butternut Squash Soup 41

Paleo Chicken Soup 44

Creamy Paleo Chicken Soup 45

Broccoli And Chicken Soup 46

Walnut And Oregano Crusted Chicken ... 49

Walnut Pesto Stuffed Chicken 50

Chicken With Olive Paste 51

Chicken And Bacon Frittata 54

Chicken And Zucchini Frittata 56

Hearty Chicken Spinach Frittata 58

Chicken And Mushroom Frittata 60

Mediterranean Chicken Stew 62

Pan Fried Liver With Bacon And Onions .. 64

Cucumber And Dried Fish Salad 66

Coconut Macaroons 67

Paleo Breakfast Sausage 69

Style Paleo Chicken Stew 71

Gutsy Granola 74

High Protein Breakfast Gold 76

Ultimate Skinny Granola 78

Scrambled Fresh Eggs With Chilli 80

Spicy Scrambled Fresh Eggs 81

Spicy India Omelet 83

Spectacular Spinach Omelet 84

Outstanding Veggie Omelette 85

Sweet Potato Hash Browns 88

Grilled Chicken 89
Cinnamon And Apple Muffins 90
Nutty Onion Scramble 92
Wholesome Porridge 93
Healthy Carrot And Sweet Potato Patties
.... 95
Banana Bread 96
Cold Chicken Salad 98
Beef And Coconut Stew 99
Soupy Chicken 100
Mango Salad With Chicken Soup 102
Watermelon And   Kiwi With Fresh Herbs
.... 105
Ginger Green Smoothie 106
Tropical Delight Fruit Bowl 107
Seasoned Seaweeds 108
Smoothie 109
Apple Chips 110
Carrot Smoothie 112

- Spicy Cauliflower 113
- Spicy Fruit Salad 114
- Kale Chips 115
- Banana Chips 116
- Fruity Cinnamon Smoothie 118
- Patrick Day Smoothie 119
- Minty Fruits Salad 120
- Blueberry And Spinach Smoothie 121
- Pumpkin Pie Spice With Sweet Potato .. 122
- Salmon, Spinach And Apple Salad 124
- Sautéed Coconut Chicken 126
- The Big Salad 127
- Paleo Pizza 129
- Macadamia Hummus With Vegetables . 132
- Carrot Soup 133
- Grilled Chicken With Olive And Tomato Topping 135
- Grilled Shrimps Salad 137

Broccoli And Pine Nuts Soup 139

Brussels Sprouts And Bacon With Tandoori Drumsticks 140

Salmon And Asparagus Salad 143

Delightful Vegetable Medley Soup........ 144

Paleo Prawns With Tomato Sauce 146

Cucumber And Watermelon Salad 148

Mushroom Cream Soup 149

Paleo Tuna Salad 151

Chicken, Tomato, Mint And Basil Salad 153

Quick And Easy Egg Salad Wrap 154

Paleo Mayonnaise Recipe 156

Sautéed Leeks With Salmon.................. 157

Chicken And Spinach 160

Lemon Grilled Chicken 161

Salmon Salad 163

Piri Piri Chicken 164

Whip Gluten-Free Banana Pancakes

Ingredients

1/2 teaspoon baking powder
4 fresh eggs
2 fresh bananas (chopped)

Procedures:

1. Place the ingredients in a bowl and mix with an immersion blender.
2. Heat a non-stick pan over medium-high heat.
3. Ladle the batter and place in the pan one at a time. Cook until the pancake bubbles, then flip and cook for another 55 seconds. Serve.

Prosciutto Wrapped Chicken

A delicious and protein rich meal.

Ingredients:

2 cups spinach (frozen, roughly chopped)
1/2 cup olives (chopped)
4 slices prosciutto
2 tbsp. olive oil
Salt and pepper to taste
4 pcs. chicken legs
2 tbsp. coconut oil
2 small shallot (chopped)
2 garlic cloves (minced)

Procedures:

1. Preheat oven to 455 °F
2. Heat the pan over medium fire and drizzle with coconut oil.
3. Sauté the garlic and shallots for 2 minutes.

4. Toss in the spinach and olives and cook for 6 minutes.
5. Remove from the heat and set in a bowl.
6. Top the mixture on the chicken thigh and wrap each leg with a slice of prosciutto.
7. Take a ceramic baking dish and drizzle with olive oil. Place the chicken on the dish and bake in the oven for an hour, or until the internal temperature reaches 356 °F.

Green Paleo Smoothie

Ingredients

1 lime (juiced)
2 pc. kiwi (diced)
2 cup coconut milk
2 pc. mango (diced)
2 cups kale (stems removed)
Water

Procedures:

1. Blend all the ingredients together, adding water to achieve your preferred consistency.

Beef Skewers And 8oz Of Water

Ingredients:

2 onion (cut into 2 " squares)
2 red or green bell pepper (cut into 2 " squares)
4 2 oz. sirloin beef (cut into 2" cubes)
2 pc. zucchini (cut into 2 " cubes)

Marinade

2 tbsp. rosemary (chopped)
1/2 cup olive oil
2 tbsp. organic tomato paste
Sea salt and pepper to taste

6 garlic cloves
2 small onion (chopped)
1/2 cup squeezed orange juice
2 tsp. orange zest

Procedures:

1. Combine all the marinade recipes in a food processor until you reach a smooth paste. Set aside 1/2 cup of the marinade for the veggies.

2. In a bowl, place beef and pour over the marinade. Toss the beef to make sure that it is well-coated with the marinade. Refrigerate it overnight.

3. When you're ready to cook, remove the beef in the fridge 55 minutes before grilling to allow it to thaw.

4. Take the it to thaw.cook, remove the beef in the fridge 55 minute

5. Thread the beef cubes and vegetables alternately using bamboo or metal skewers.

6. Bring the grill over medium heat and cook the kebabs, turning each side after four minutes. The whole kebab will cook in about 28 minutes.

Breakfast Paleo Waffles

Ingredients:

1/2 teaspoon salt

4 fresh eggs , separated

35 ml (2 tablespoon) olive oil

1/2 cup coconut milk

2 cup almond flour

55 ml (2 tablespoons) coconut flour

1 teaspoon baking soda

1/2 teaspoon cinnamon

1/2 cup unsweetened organic applesauce or mashed ripe banana (depends on your taste)

2 teaspoon vanilla

Fresh fruits for garnish or unsweetened organic applesauce or maple syrup

Instructions:

1. Lightly grease the waffle maker with coconut butter and preheat.
2. In a bowl, beat egg whites on high speed for about 4 minutes, until they form stiff peaks.
3. In a bowl, mix flour, baking soda, cinnamon, and salt. In another bowl, whisk egg yolks, milk, apple sauce, or mashed banana, vanilla and oil.
4. Add flour mixture to the wet mixture and combine well. Fold in 1/2 of the egg whites and mix well.
5. Add another 1/2 of egg whites, and gently fold it into the batter.
6. Repeat twice. You should have a light and fluffy batter.
7. Place ⅓ cup to 1 cup of the batter in the greased waffle iron. Close gently and cook until golden browned.

8. Top with fresh fruits or unsweetened organic applesauce or a maple syrup drizzle

Hungry Man Steak And Bacon Hash

Ingredients:

1 cup green bell pepper chopped

1 cup red bell pepper, chopped

2 sweet potato, cubed

2 zucchini, cubed

2 garlic cloves, minced

2 tablespoon jalapeños pepper, minced

4 paleo-approved bacon strips, chopped

1 pound of thinly sliced beef strips such as sirloin, chopped

4 fresh eggs

2 tablespoons olive oil (optional)

1 cup chopped onions

Sea salt and fresh ground pepper to taste

Instructions:

1. Pre-heat the oven at 200ºC/400 F
2. In a fresh frying pan, cook the bacon for 2-4 minutes until golden on high heat.
3. Add onions and garlic, and continue cooking on medium heat for 2-4 minutes.
4. Add the beef and sweet potatoes, cook for 5-10 minutes until the meat is cooked.
5. Add remaining ingredients and cook for an additional 25 minutes or until all the vegetables are tender. Season with salt and pepper to taste.
6. Remove the pan from heat.

7. In another frying pan, cook the fresh eggs sunny side up until done.
8. Season with salt and pepper to taste
9. Spoon 1/2 of the meat and vegetables mix on a plate, top with one sunny egg. Repeat for each serving.

No-Crust Mini Bacon Quiches

Ingredients:

2 tablespoons olive oil (optional)

1 cup chopped onions

1 cup green bell pepper chopped

1 cup red bell pepper, chopped

4 paleo-approved bacon strips, chopped

6 fresh eggs

Sea salt and fresh ground pepper to taste

Coconut butter or olive oil for greasing

Paprika to sprinkle

Instructions:

1. Pre-heat the oven at 2 10 0ºC/490 Fº.
2. In a fresh frying pan, cook the bacon for 10 minutes until golden brown on medium-high heat. Add onions, cooking on medium heat for 2 minutes. Add peppers, cook for 2 minutes, season with salt and pepper to taste. Remove the pan from heat and let cool a few minutes.
3. In the meantime, whisk the fresh eggs vigorously for 2-4 minutes until very fluffy, then add the vegetables and bacon to the fresh eggs and combine well. . Season with salt and pepper to taste.

4. Grease generously a muffin pan with olive oil or coconut butter. Fill ¾ of each muffin hole with the egg mixture
5. Bake the egg muffins in the pre-heated oven for 2 0-28 minutes or until golden brown. Let cool for 6 -25 minutes before unmolding, sprinkle with paprika.
6. Serve hot with slices of tomatoes.

Pumpkin Breakfast Pancakes

Ingredients:

- 6 ml (2 teaspoon) pumpkin pie spice
- 6 ml (2 teaspoon) cinnamon
- 6 ml (2 teaspoon) vanilla extract
- 2 fresh eggs , lightly beaten
- 35 ml (2 tablespoon) toasted almonds, chopped
- 35 ml (2 tablespoon) maple syrup

- 55 ml (2 teaspoons) coconut oil
- 280 ml (2 cup) pumpkin, pre-boiled and mashed
- 35 ml (2 tablespoon) almond butter

Directions:

1. Mash pumpkin in a bowl. Mix with almond butter.
2. Add in pumpkin pie spice, cinnamon and vanilla extract and mix well.
3. Stir in fresh eggs and whisk to combine well.
4. Heat oil in a nonstick skillet on medium heat.
5. Add 4 heaping tablespoons of batter into the pan and cook pancake for 2-4 minutes or until nicely golden. Flip and cook the other side and repeat until all batter is gone.

6. Serve on a plate, sprinkled with toasted nuts and drizzled with maple syrup.

Poblano Pepper Omelet

Ingredients:

- 2 poblano pepper, sliced
- 2 fresh onion, chopped
- 2 tomato, chopped
- Salt and pepper to taste
- 55 ml (2 tablespoons) coconut oil
- 4 fresh eggs
- 2 avocado, sliced

Directions:

1. Crack fresh eggs in a bowl, season with salt and pepper and whisk.
2. Heat oil in a frying pan.
3. Pour fresh eggs in the pan. Tilt the pan to spread the fresh eggs evenly. Top with avocado slices, poblano pepper, onion and tomato.
4. Cook for 10 minutes or until set and slightly golden. Flip and cook the other side for 6 more minutes or until lightly golden. Fold into half and serve on a plate.

Jalapeño Scrambled Fresh Eggs With Cherry Tomatoes

Ingredients:

- 46 ml (4 tablespoons) almond butter
- 280 ml (2 cup) cherry tomatoes, halved
- 2 small jalapeños, seeded and chopped

- 4 scallions, chopped
- 4 fresh fresh eggs
- 2 egg whites
- Salt and black pepper, to taste
- 6 ml (2 teaspoon) dried thyme

Directions

1. In a bowl, add fresh eggs , egg whites, salt, black pepper and thyme and whisk well.
2. Melt butter in a frying pan over medium high heat.
3. Add tomatoes and jalapeños, and cook for 2 to 4 minutes.
4. Add egg mixture and cook for 4 to 10 minutes until fresh eggs are done completely, stirring occasionally.
5. Stir in scallions and cook for 5 to 10 minutes.

Peachy Pancakes

Ingredients:

- 55 ml (2 tablespoons) coconut flour
- 46 ml (4 tablespoons) ground flax seed
- Pinch of cinnamon
- Pinch of salt
- 55 ml (2 tablespoons) coconut oil
- 280 ml (2 cup) peaches, chopped
- 2 fresh eggs
- 75 ml (1/2 cup) coconut milk
- 2 ml (1/2 teaspoon) vanilla extract
- 35 ml (2 tablespoon) ground almond

Directions

1. Lightly whisk fresh eggs in a bowl, and add peaches.
2. Mix in coconut milk and vanilla extract and continue whisking.

3. In another bowl, mix together ground almond, coconut flour, flax seed, cinnamon, and salt.
4. Gradually add this mixture into fresh eggs , and combine well using a fork.
5. Heat coconut oil in a nonstick frying pan. Spoon 55 ml (2 tablespoons) of this batter into the pan and flatten it using backside of spoon.
6. Cook for 2-4 minutes or until slightly golden. Flip and cook other side, and repeat until all batter is gone. Serve in a plate topped with peach slices.

Mexican Scramble

Ingredients:

- 270 ml (1 cup) tomatoes, chopped
- 6 ml (2 teaspoon) cumin
- 2 fresh fresh eggs
- Seasons with salt and pepper
- 55 ml (2 tablespoons) parsley, chopped

- 55 ml (2 tablespoons) coconut oil
- 2 medium fresh onion, chopped
- 6 cloves garlic, minced
- 2 red bell pepper, deseeded, julienne
- 2 jalapeño pepper, deseeded, julienne

Directions:

1. Heat oil in a fresh frying pan.
2. Stir in onion and garlic and cook for few minutes until little browned.
3. Add red bell pepper, jalapeño and tomatoes and continue to cook until the vegetables are tender.
4. Sprinkle with cumin and salt.
5. Crack fresh eggs in a bowl and season with salt and pepper.
6. Pour fresh eggs in the frying pan.
7. Cook for 10 minutes or until slightly golden. Flip and cook other side until fresh eggs are done.

8. Sprinkle with parsley and serve.

Healthy Granola Bars

Ingredients:

55 ml (2 tablespoons) sunflower seeds

55 ml (2 tablespoons) sesame seeds

55 ml (2 tablespoons) almonds, sliced

75 ml (4 tablespoons) freshly squeezed orange juice

35 ml (2 tablespoon) coconut oil

55 ml (2 tablespoons) raw honey

55 ml (2 tablespoons) pumpkin seeds

55 ml (2 tablespoons) poppy seeds

Directions:

1. Preheat oven to 2 80ºC/4 6 0°F. Lightly grease a baking dish with olive oil.
2. Combine all ingredients in a bowl and seasons with salt and pepper.
3. Spread batter over a baking dish.
4. Bake for 25 to 35 minutes or until golden browned. Remove from oven and let it cool.
5. Cut into bars and refrigerate for at least 2 hour until set before serving.

Paleo Beef Jerky

Ingredients:

3 ml (1 teaspoon) chipotle powder

3 ml (1 teaspoon) onion powder

3 ml (1 teaspoon) ginger powder

3 ml (1 teaspoon) salt

3 ml (1 teaspoon) black pepper

235 g (1 pound) flank steak

55 ml (2 tablespoons) Coconut Amino

2 garlic clove, mined

3 ml (1 teaspoon) smoked paprika

Directions:

1. Preheat the oven to 60ºC/2 8 0°F. Lightly grease a baking dish.
2. Combine all ingredients in a bowl and mix together.
3. Leave marinated for at least 2 hours or overnight.
4. Put stake on the baking dish and bake for 4 to 4 hours.

Spicy Nuts

Ingredients:

75 ml (1/2 cup) walnuts, toasted

3 ml (1 teaspoon) chili powder

2 ml (1/2 teaspoon) cumin

Pinch of salt and pepper

6 ml (2 teaspoon) coconut oil

75 ml (1/2 cup) pecans, toasted

75 ml (1/2 cup) almonds, toasted

Directions:

1. Toss all ingredients in a mixing bowl and season with salt and pepper.

4 slices of ham
2 fresh eggs
(spices for flavor)

Procedures:

1. Preheat your oven to 400°F
2. Prepare a muffin pan by greasing it with coconut oil.
3. Place two pieces of ham on top of each other in one muffin cup. Repeat with the next muffin cup.
4. Crack the egg on top of the ham
a. *(Optional: add scallions, basil, etc. on your egg for more flavor)*
5. Bake for 35 minutes and serve.

Veggie-Bun Sandwich

Ingredients:

1 avocado (cut into strips)
2 pc. seaweed strips
2 pc. red bell pepper
2 slices turkey ham

Procedures:

1. Take the bell pepper and slice it in half and remove the seeds.
2. Take one piece of bell pepper and top it with the ham, seaweed, and avocado.
3. Top with the other half of the bell pepper and stick a toothpick in the center.
4. Enjoy.

Low-Carb Paleo Patties And 8oz Of Water

Ingredients:

a pinch of cayenne pepper
a pinch of salt
a pinch of ground pepper
2 pcs. green onions (chopped)
2 pc. tomato (sliced)
2 cups arugula
2 pc. avocado (sliced)
35 oz. ground lean turkey
2 tsp. paprika
1 tsp. coriander
2 tsp. powdered onion

Procedures:

1. In a bowl, place the ground turkey and add the onion powder, salt, pepper, paprika, cayenne pepper, and green onions and combine everything.

2. Use your hands to form into burger patties.

3. Heat the grill and cook the burgers for 6 minutes, per side.

4. Place the cooked patties over the arugula, tomatoes, and avocado. Serve.

Walnut Pesto Chicken Salad

2 fresh apple, peeled and diced

2 fresh avocado, peeled and diced

2 cups cooked chicken, diced

for the walnut pesto

2-4 green olives

4 tbsps extra virgin olive oil

2 tbsp lemon juice

salt and black pepper, to taste

1 cup walnuts, chopped

25 fresh basil leaves

2 garlic clove

Directions:

1. In a food processor, blend together walnuts, olives, basil, olive oil, garlic and lemon juice until completely smooth.
2. Combine diced chicken, apple, and avocado. Pour over the walnut pesto, stir to combine and serve.

Grilled Chicken Salad

Ingredients:

2 red bell pepper, sliced

4 -4 green onions, chopped

2 tbsp balsamic vinegar

2 tsp dried oregano

2 cups grilled chicken breasts, diced

1/2 cup black olives, pitted

2 cup grape tomatoes

2 tbsp extra virgin olive oil

Salt and black pepper, to taste

Directions:

1. Place chicken in a deep salad bowl. Add in the grape tomatoes, fresh onion, red pepper and olives. Season with salt and pepper.
2. Toss gently to combine, sprinkle with oregano, balsamic vinegar and olive oil, and serve.

Chicken And Broccoli Salad

2 garlic cloves, crushed

2 tsp dried basil

2 tbsp extra virgin olive oil

4 tbsp balsamic vinegar

1 tsp salt

2 cooked chicken breasts, diced

2 small head broccoli, cut into florets

2 cup cherry tomatoes, halved

Directions:

1. Heat two tablespoons of olive oil in a non-stick frying pan and gently sauté broccoli for 5-10 minutes until tender. Add in garlic and basil and cook for one minute.
2. Place broccoli in a fresh salad bowl. Stir in the chicken and tomatoes. Season with salt and sprinkle with vinegar and

remaining olive oil. Toss to combine and serve.

Vitamin Chicken Salad

2 small green apple, peeled and thinly sliced

1 cup toasted almonds, chopped

4 tbsp lemon juice

2 tbsp extra virgin olive oil

2 tbsp Dijon mustard

salt and pepper, to taste

4 cooked chicken breasts, shredded

2 yellow bell pepper, thinly sliced

2 red bell pepper, thinly sliced

2 small red fresh onion, thinly sliced

Directions:

1. In a deep salad bowl, combine peppers, apple, chicken and almonds.
2. In a smaller bowl, whisk the mustard, olive oil, lemon juice, salt and pepper.
3. Pour over the salad, toss to combine and serve.

Chicken, Lettuce And Avocado Salad

5-10 radishes, sliced

8 -8 grape tomatoes, halved

4 tbsp lemon juice

4 tbsp extra virgin olive oil

2 tsp dried mint

2 grilled chicken breasts, diced

2 avocado, peeled and diced

5-10 green lettuce leaves, cut in stripes

4 -4 green onions, finely chopped

salt and black pepper, to taste

Directions:

1. In a deep salad bowl, combine avocados, lettuce, chicken, onions, radishes and grape tomatoes. Season with mint, salt and pepper to taste. Sprinkle with lemon juice and olive oil. Toss lightly and serve.

Mashed Avocado And Chicken Salad

4 tbsp lemon juice

2 tbsp extra virgin olive oil

2 tbsp fresh taragon leaves, finely cut

salt and pepper, to taste

2 cooked chicken breasts, diced

2 small red fresh onion, finely chopped

2 ripe avocados, mashed with a fork

Directions:

1. Place the chicken in a medium sized salad bowl. In a plate, mash the avocados using either a fork or a potato masher and add them to the chicken.
2. Add in the fresh onion, taragon, lemon juice and olive oil. Season with salt and black pepper to taste, stir to combine and serve.

Easy Chicken And Egg Salad

1 cup walnuts, roasted

2 tbsp lemon juice

2 tbsp extra virgin olive oil

salt and pepper, to taste

2 cups cooked chicken, chopped

2 hard boiled fresh eggs , diced

a bunch of arugula leaves

2 fresh apple, diced

Directions:

1. Roast walnuts in a preheated to 46 0 F oven for 2-4 minutes or until toasted.
2. In a deep salad bowl, combine chicken, apple, fresh eggs and arugula. In a smaller bowl, whisk lemon juice, olive oil, salt and black pepper. Pour over the chicken mixture. Top with walnuts and serve.

Mediterranean Chicken Soup

2 bay leaf

6 cups water

6-8 black olives, pitted and halved

1 tsp salt

black pepper, to taste

fresh parsley, to serve

lemon juice, to serve

4 chicken breasts

2 carrot, chopped

2 small zucchini, peeled and chopped

2 celery rib, chopped

2 small fresh onion, chopped

Directions:

1. Place chicken breasts, fresh onion, carrot, celery and bay leaf in a deep soup pot.

2. Add in salt, black pepper and 6 cups of water.
3. Stir well and bring to a boil. Add zucchini and olives and reduce heat.
4. Simmer for 55 minutes.
5. Remove chicken from the pot and set aside to cool.
6. Shred it and return it back to the pot.
7. Serve with lemon juice and sprinkled with parsley.

Chicken And Butternut Squash Soup

6 cups water

1/2 tsp cumin

2 tbsp paprika

4 tbsp extra virgin olive oil

4 boneless chicken thighs, diced

1 fresh onion, chopped

6-8 white mushrooms, chopped

2 small zucchini, peeled and diced

2 cup butternut squash, diced

2 tbsp tomato paste

Directions:

1. In a deep soup pot, heat olive oil and gently sauté fresh onion, stirring occasionally.
2. Add chicken and cook for 2-4 minutes.
3. Stir in cumin, paprika and butternut squash.
4. Dilute the tomato paste in a cup of water and add to the soup.
5. Add in the remaining water and bring to a boil.
6. Reduce heat and simmer for 25 minutes then add zucchini and mushrooms.
7. Simmer until butternut squash is tender.
8. Season with salt and black pepper to taste.

Paleo Chicken Soup

2 red bell pepper, chopped

2 celery rib, chopped

2 bay leaf

2 tsp salt

1 cup fresh parsley leaves, finely cut

black pepper, to taste

4 boneless chicken tights, chopped

2 small fresh onion, chopped

4 garlic cloves

2 sweet potato, skinned and diced

2 fresh carrot, chopped

Directions:

1. Place the chicken, bay leaf, celery, carrot, fresh onion, red pepper, sweet

potato and salt into a pot with 6 cups of cold water.
2. Bring to the boil, reduce heat and simmer for 55 minutes.
3. Season with salt and pepper, add in parsley, simmer for 2-4 minutes and serve.

Creamy Paleo Chicken Soup

2 celery rib, chopped

2 small fresh onion, chopped

6 cups water

1 tsp salt

4 chicken breasts

2 carrot, chopped

2 cup zucchini, peeled and chopped

2 cups cauliflower, broken into florets

black pepper, to taste

Directions:

1. Place chicken breasts, fresh onion, carrot, celery, cauliflower and zucchini in a deep soup pot.
2. Add in salt, black pepper and 6 cups of water. Stir and bring to a boil.
3. Simmer for 55 minutes then remove chicken from the pot and let it cool slightly.
4. Blend soup until completely smooth.
5. Shred or dice the chicken meat, return it back to the pot, stir and serve.

Broccoli And Chicken Soup

2 garlic clove, chopped

2 small fresh onion, chopped

4 cups water

4 tbsp extra virgin olive oil

1 tsp salt

4 boneless chicken thighs, diced

2 small carrot, chopped

2 broccoli head, broken into florets

black pepper, to taste

Directions:

1. In a deep soup pot, heat olive oil and gently sauté broccoli for 2-4 minutes, stirring occasionally.
2. Add in fresh onion, carrot, chicken and cook, stirring, for 2-4 minutes.
3. Stir in the salt, black pepper and water.
4. Bring to a boil.
5. Simmer for 55 minutes then remove from heat and set aside to cool.
6. In a blender or food processor, blend soup until completely smooth.
7. Serve and enjoy!

Walnut And Oregano Crusted Chicken

1 cup walnuts, chopped

2 garlic cloves, chopped

2 fresh eggs , beaten

4 skinless, boneless chicken breasts

2 0-28 fresh oregano leaves

salt and pepper,to taste

Directions:

1. Blend the garlic, oregano and walnuts in a food processor until a rough crumb is formed.
2. Season with salt and black pepper.
3. Stir and place this mixture on a plate.
4. Whisk fresh eggs in a deep bowl.
5. Dip each chicken breast in the beaten egg then roll it in the walnut mixture.

6. Place coated chicken on a baking tray and bake at 490 F for 2 4 minutes each side.

Walnut Pesto Stuffed Chicken

2 tbsp chia seeds

2-4 green olives

4 tbsps extra virgin olive oil

2 tbsp lemon juice

4 fresh chicken breasts

1 cup walnuts, chopped

25 fresh basil leaves

2 garlic clove

salt and black pepper, to taste

Directions:

1. In a food processor, blend together walnuts, olives, basil, olive oil, garlic, chia

seeds and lemon juice until completely smooth.
2. Carefully butterfly each chicken breast.
3. Cover with plastic wrap and beat with a heavy object until the breast is flattened.
4. Put a tablespoon of the walnut mixture in each breast and roll over the top part like a flap.
5. Season with salt and black pepper and bake at 490 F for 4 6 minutes.

Chicken With Olive Paste

2 garlic cloves, crushed

2 chicken breasts (each cut into 2 cutlets)

for the olive paste:

2 tbsp tomato paste

2 tbsp basil, chopped

4 tbsp extra virgin olive oil

salt and pepper, to taste

2 tbsp olive oil

- 2 cloves garlic, peeled
- 1/2 cup pitted black olives
- 2 tbsp capers

Directions:

1. Place the garlic cloves into a food processor together with the olives, capers, basil, tomato paste and olive oil.
2. Blend until smooth. Season to taste with salt and pepper.
3. Gently heat oil in a skillet on medium heat. Add in the chicken cutlets and cook each side for 4-6 minutes.
4. Serve each cutlet topped with olive paste.

Chicken And Bacon Frittata

Ingredients:

2 red bell pepper, diced

2 small tomato, diced

4 fresh eggs whisked

4 tbsp coconut milk

1 tsp dried oregano

1 tsp dried parsley

4 tbsp olive oil

1 cup chicken, chopped finely

4 oz bacon, chopped

4-6 green onions, finely chopped

2 garlic clove, chopped

Directions:

1. Heat two tablespoons of olive oil in a frying pan and gently cook the chicken until almost cooked through.

2. Add the onions and garlic and cook for another minute. Set aside.
3. In the same pan, heat the remaining olive oil.
4. Cook the bell pepper and tomato for 2-4 minutes, until lightly cooked.
5. Add in the chicken, bacon and green onions, and mix well. Pour it all into a baking dish.
6. In a medium bowl, whisk fresh eggs , coconut milk and seasonings together.
7. Pour over the top of the meat and vegetable mixture, making sure that it covers it well.
8. Bake in a preheated to 4 75 F oven for about 35 minutes, or until fresh eggs are cooked through.

Chicken And Zucchini Frittata

2 tomato, diced

2 tbsp dill, finely chopped

4 fresh eggs

4 tbsp coconut milk

4 tbsp olive oil

2 cup chicken, chopped finely

1 fresh onion, finely chopped

2 garlic cloves, chopped

2 zucchini, peeled and diced

1. Heat two tablespoons of olive oil in a frying pan and gently cook the chicken until almost cooked through.
2. Add the onion and garlic and cook for another minute. Set aside.
3. In the same pan, heat the remaining olive oil. Cook the zucchini and tomato for for 4 -4 minutes, until lightly cooked.

4. Add in the chicken and mix everything well. Pour it all into the baking dish.
5. In a medium bowl, whisk fresh eggs , coconut milk and dill together.
6. Pour over the top of the chicken and vegetable mixture, making sure that it covers it well.
7. Bake in a preheated to 4 75 F oven for around 35 minutes, until set.
8. Garnish with fresh dill.

Hearty Chicken Spinach Frittata

1 zucchini, peeled and shredded

2 fresh tomato, thinly sliced

2 tbsp fresh rosemary leaves, finely chopped

6 fresh eggs

4 tbsp coconut milk

4 tbsp olive oil

2 cup chicken, chopped finely

4 -4 green onions, finely chopped

6 oz frozen chopped spinach, defrosted and excess moisture squeezed out

Directions:

1. Grease a shallow casserole dish.
2. Heat two tablespoons of olive oil in a frying pan and gently cook the chicken until almost cooked through.

3. Add in the onions and garlic and cook for another minute. Set aside.
4. In the same pan, heat the remaining olive oil.
5. Cook the zucchini and spinach, stirring constantly, until lightly cooked.
6. Add in the chicken mixture, and combine everything well.
7. Pour it all into the casserole.
8. In a medium bowl, whisk fresh eggs , coconut milk and rosemary together.
9. Pour over the top of the chicken and vegetable mixture, making sure that it covers it well.
10. Lay the tomato slices on top. Bake in a preheated to 4 /5 F oven for around 35 minutes, until set.
11. Garnish with rosemary.

Chicken And Mushroom Frittata

1 tsp salt

1 tsp black pepper

2 tsp dried thyme

4 fresh fresh eggs , beaten well

2 tbsp extra virgin olive oil

2 cup roasted chicken meat, chopped

2 cup white mushrooms, chopped

1 fresh onion, chopped

2 garlic cloves, chopped

2 fresh tomato, thinly sliced

Directions:

1. Grease a shallow casserole dish.
2. Heat two tablespoons of olive oil in a frying pan and gently cook the onions and garlic until onion is transparent.
3. Add in the mushrooms, stir, and cook on medium-high heat for 4 -4 minutes.

4. Add in the chicken and combine everything well.
5. Pour it into the casserole.
6. In a medium bowl, whisk fresh eggs , coconut milk, salt, black pepper and thyme together.
7. Pour over the top of the chicken and mushroom mixture, making sure that it covers it well.
8. Lay the tomato slices on top.
9. Bake in a preheated to 4 75 F oven for around 35 minutes, until set.

Mediterranean Chicken Stew

2 cup tomato sauce

2 cup assorted olives, pitted

2 tsp dried basil

1 cup fresh parsley, finely chopped

4 tbsp extra virgin olive oil

4 chicken breasts

2 fresh onion, chopped

2 small zucchini, peeled and chopped

2 red bell pepper, chopped

Directions:

1. In a deep pan, heat olive oil and seal the chicken breasts.
2. Set aside in a plate.
3. In the same pan, gently sauté the onion and bell pepper, stirring, for 2-4 minutes, or until the onion has softened.
4. Return chicken to the pan.

5. Add in zucchini, tomato sauce, olives, basil, salt and pepper.
6. Cover the pan and bring to a boil. Reduce heat and simmer for 55 minutes, or until the chicken is cooked through.
7. Sprinkle with fresh parsley and serve.

Pan Fried Liver With Bacon And Onions

Ingredients

- 2 2-35   almonds

- Paprika or crushed black pepper per taste

- 1/2 tsp. nutmeg powder

- Salt per taste

- 2 tbsps. Ghee

- 2 tbsps. Lightly chopped cilantro

- 3-5 piece bacon

- 2 fresh onion, large, chopped

- 2 small liver (turkey or chicken)

- 2 tbsp. coconut oil

Instructions

1. Roast bacon lightly in a frying pan on medium heat. Keep aside when done.
2. In another pan stir fry onion slices in 2 tbsp. coconut oil over medium heat.
3. Add salt and pepper per taste. Sauté for 20-35 minutes or till the onions get caramelized fully. Keep aside.
4. Pulse almonds until a flour like consistency is achieved. You can also use pre-made almond flour.
5. In a bowl add the almond flour, paprika or pepper, salt and nutmeg. Mix well.
6. Rinse and pat dry the liver and make about 1 inch slices.
7. In another pan heat ghee.
8. Dredge the liver slices in the almond flour carefully.
9. Make sure to coat it well.
10. Stir-fry the liver slices in ghee for about two minutes on each side.
11. To serve place the hot liver slices on a dish and top them with the onions.
12. Put the bacon slices over the onions and garnish with cilantro or parsley.

Cucumber And Dried Fish Salad

Ingredients

- 2 tbsps. Apple cider vinegar (lime juice can be used as well)
- Salt to taste
- Sesame seeds for garnish
- ¾ cups dried fish
- 4 medium cucumbers, chopped thinly
- 6 tbsps. Olive oil (sesame oil can be used as well)

Instructions

1. Take a fresh mixing bowl and add all the ingredients one by one.
2. Toss well.
3. While serving add more dressing if needed.

Coconut Macaroons

Ingredients

- 1 tsp ginger, chopped
- 2 cups coconut flakes
- 2 tbsps. Coconut cream
- Coconut oil for greasing
- 1 cup walnuts, soaked
- 2 small cup dates, seeded and roughly chopped
- Vanilla Extract

Instructions

1. Keep the oven on preheat mode at 4 6 0 F for 25 minutes.
2. In a mixing bowl add walnuts, ginger, vanilla extract and ginger and mix well. Pulse this mixture in a food processor. Remove and keep aside.

3. Add coconut cream and coconut flakes to the food processor and pulse.
4. Now add the above mixture to the food processor and pulse till all the ingredients are combined. Remove in a bowl.
5. Knead the mixture with your hands and keep aside.
6. Take a baking dish and grease it lightly with the coconut oil.
7. Grease your palms lightly as well.
8. Make small cookie sized balls and flatten them on the baking dish. Remember these will not change shape after baking!
9. Bake for 26 -55 minutes at 4 6 0 F.

Paleo Breakfast Sausage

Ingredients

- 4 tbsp maple syrup
- 4 tbsp lemon juice
- Salt to taste
- Pepper, freshly ground
- Cayenne, to taste
- Red chili flakes
- 4 lbs. pork, ground
- 4 tsp. sage, lightly crushed
- 4 -6 cloves garlic, lightly crushed
- 4 green onions, chopped roughly

Instructions

1. Take a fresh mixing bowl and add all the ingredients one by one while keeping the pork aside.
2. Mix everything well until combined properly.
3. Add pork to the above mixture and mix well.
4. Grease your palms lightly with any Paleo friendly oil and make small patties of the pork mixture.
5. Heat a fresh frying pan on medium heat and brown the patties on both the sides.
6. Serve hot with your favorite dip.

Style Paleo Chicken Stew

Ingredients

- 4-6 cloves garlic, minced
- 2 1/2 tbsp garam masala
- Cayenne, to taste
- 4 tsp cumin
- 1 tsp coriander powder
- 28 /2 cups homemade chicken broth
- 1/2 cup coconut cream
- 2 cup tomato puree
- 2 sweet potatoes, small, peeled and diced
- Cilantro, for garnish
- 2 tbsp coconut oil, divided
- 2 chicken breasts, boneless
- Salt, to taste

- Ground pepper, fresh
- 2 yellow fresh onion, chopped
- 2 inch piece of ginger, minced

Instructions

1. Marinate chicken for 25 minutes by coating it with generous amount of salt and pepper.
2. Take a Dutch oven and heat 2 tbsp coconut oil in it on medium.
3. Place the chicken in the oven and let it brown in each side for five minutes.
4. Generously season the chicken with salt and pepper and place into the pan.
5. Brown on each side for 4-6 minutes. Remove and keep aside.
6. In the same oven add the rest of the oil and heat it on medium heat again.
7. When hot enough add garlic, onions and ginger. Sauté for 6 -8 minutes till the onions become translucent.

8. Once onions become soft enough, add cumin, garam masala, coriander and cayenne along with one tbsp of tomato puree. Mix well and let it simmer for 4-6 minutes.
9. Add broth, chicken breasts and all the remaining puree to the pot.
10. Let it boil and. then reduce the heat. Let it cook with a lid on for about 4 hours on low to medium heat.
11. Take off the lid after 4 hours season the stew with salt and pepper.
12. Take out all the chicken pieces and shred them lightly.
13. Re-add the chicken along with the sweet potato to the pot and let cook for around 4 0-40 minutes with lid closed. Stir occasionally.

Gutsy Granola

Ingredients:

- 1/2 cup sunflower seeds, shelled
- 1 cup unsweetened coconut flakes
- 1/2 cup coconut oil
- Stevia to taste
- 2 tsp vanilla
- low sodium salt to taste
- 2 cup cashews
- 1/3 cup almonds
- 1/2 cup pumpkin seeds, shelled

Instructions:

1. Preheat oven to 455 degrees F. Line a baking sheet with parchment paper.
2. Place the cashews, almonds, coconut flakes and pumpkin seeds into a blender and pulse to break the mixture into smaller pieces.

3. In a fresh microwave-safe bowl, melt the coconut oil, vanilla, and stevia together for 40-6 0 seconds.
4. Add in the mixture from the blender and the sunflower seeds, and stir to coat.
5. Spread the mixture out onto the baking sheet and cook for 20-26 minutes, stirring once, until the mixture is lightly browned. Remove from heat. Add low sodium salt.
6. Press the granola mixture together to form a flat, even surface.
7. Cool for about 35 minutes, and then break into pieces.

High Protein Breakfast Gold

Ingredients:

- 2 tbs. dark ground cinnamon
- 2 tbs. hemp protein powder
- 2 tbs. coconut oil, melted
- 1 cup (c). Flax-Meal, golden
- 1 c. Chia seed
- Stevia liquid to taste

Instructions:

1. Begin to spread the dough out until its super thin, onto a parchment paper lined cookie sheet.
2. Bake at 455 for 35 minutes, then drop it down to 455 and leave for 55 minutes.
3. Before dropping it, pull out the sheet and cut it.

4. Put it back into the oven exactly like this, don't separate the pieces.
5. When the 55 minutes are up, pull it out and separate the pieces.
6. Drop the pieces to 270 degrees F for 2 hour. They will be completely dried out at this point.

Enjoy with almond or other nut milk!

Ultimate Skinny Granola

Ingredients:

2 cup of unsweetened coconut milk or unsweetened almond milk

Stevia liquid to taste
2 tablespoon each of unsalted ...

pecan pieces
walnut pieces
almonds
pistachios
raw pine nuts
raw sunflower/safflower seeds
raw pumpkin seeds
2 Tablespoons of frozen or fresh berry selection (e.g. blueberries, blackberries, raspberries, strawberries, or other kinds etc)

Instructions:

1. Put all the nuts and seeds in a breakfast bowl.
2. add a few drops of pure liquid stevia and stir it well in.
3. Add the berries and milk.
4. If using frozen berries, wait for 2-4 minutes for them to get warmer.
5. The berries will now release some color into the milk, making it look really interesting.

Scrambled Fresh Eggs With Chilli

Ingredients:

- 4 fresh green chillies with skins removed
- 2 tablespoons (4 0g or 2 oz) coconut oil
- 2 small fresh onion, peeled and finely chopped
- 6 fresh eggs
- 1/2 cup (62ml or 2 fl oz) coconut milk
- low sodium salt to taste

Instructions:

1. After removing chilli skins, remove and discard seeds and finely chop remaining chilli.
2. Beat fresh eggs , coconut milk and salt in a bowl and set aside.
3. Heat oil in a medium size saucepan over a medium heat.

4. Reduce heat to low and add egg mixture to saucepan and mix well.
5. Scatter chilies over mixture.
6. Cook over a low heat until fresh eggs are cooked.
7. Serves 4. Serve hot.

Spicy Scrambled Fresh Eggs

Ingredients:

- 2 chilli, seeded and cut into thin strips
- 4 ripe tomatoes, peeled, seeded, and chopped
- Salt and freshly ground black pepper
- 4 fresh organic fresh eggs
- 2 tablespoon extra-virgin olive oil
- 2 red fresh onion, finely chopped

- 2 medium green pepper, cored, seeded, and finely chopped

Instructions:

1. Heat the olive oil in a large, heavy, preferably nonstick skillet over medium heat.
2. Add the onion and cook until soft, 6 to 8 minutes.
3. Add the pepper and chilli and continue cooking until soft, another 4 to 6 minutes.
4. Add in the tomatoes, and salt and pepper to taste and cook uncovered, over low heat for 25 minutes.
5. Add the fresh eggs , stirring them into the mixture to distribute.
6. Cover the skillet and cook until the fresh eggs are set but still fluffy and tender, about 8 to 8 minutes. Divide between 4 plates and serve.

Spicy India Omelet

Ingredients:

4 Green Chilli (optional)

1/2 cup Coconut grated

Low sodium Salt as required

2 tblspoon olive oil

4 Fresh eggs

2 Fresh onion, chopped

Instructions:
1. Beat the Fresh eggs severely.
2. Mix chopped fresh onion, rounded green chilli, salt and grated coconuts with fresh eggs .
3. Heat oil on a medium-low heat, in a pan.

4. Pour the mixture in the form of pancakes and cook it on the both sides.

Spectacular Spinach Omelet

Ingredients:

- coconut oil, about 2 tbsp
- 1/2 c tomatoes and onion salsa (lightly fried in pan)
- 2 tbsp fresh cilantro
- 2 fresh eggs
- 3 cups raw spinach

Instructions:

1. Melt coconut oil on medium in frying pan.
2. Add spinach, cook until mostly wilted. Beat fresh eggs and add to pan.
3. Flip once the egg sets around the edge.

4. When it's almost done add the salsa on top just to warm it.
5. Move to plate and add cilantro. Serves one.

Outstanding Veggie Omelette

Ingredients:

- 2   handful tiny broccoli florets or whatever leftover veggies you have
- Bits of leftover cooked turkey
- Safflower oil
- Low sodium salt
- 4 fresh eggs , beaten
- 2 carrot, matchstick cut
- 4 scallions, diagonal sliced

Instructions:

1. Heat oil in a wok or fresh cast iron skillet over medium heat, until hot enough to sizzle a drop of water.
2. Add broccoli and carrots, stir fry 2 min. until soft.
3. Add cooked turkey, stir fry 2 min. until heated through.
4. Add scallions and fresh eggs , scramble.
5. Add salt to taste. Serve.

Sweet Potato Hash Browns

Serves- 2
Ingredients

- 2-4 Sweet potatoes
- Oil of choice (from foods you can eat list).
- 1 teaspoon Allspice powder
- 2 medium chopped onion (optional)
- Salt to taste
- Pepper to taste

Directions

1. Grate the sweet potatoes with the help of a cheese grater into a bowl.
2. Season with allspice powder, salt and pepper.
3. Add the chopped onions and mix.

4. Heat a medium frying pan and pour oil into it.
5. Add the sweet potato mixture and cook on medium low flame.
6. When light golden brown, flip and cook on the other side.
7. Serve hot.

Grilled Chicken

Serves: 2
Ingredients

- 2 tablespoon olive oil
- 2 teaspoon turmeric powder
- 2 teaspoon cumin powder
- 1 teaspoon cinnamon powder
- 2 fresh garlic clove
- 2 diced chicken breasts
- 2 tablespoons lemon juice
- 2 teaspoons raw honey
- Salt to taste
- Pepper to taste

Directions

1. Make a marinade by combining together, in a bowl, garlic, cumin, cinnamon, turmeric and olive oil.
2. Add the diced chicken to this mixture. Keep in the fridge for about thirty minutes to marinate.
3. Preheat the grill to 4 6 0°F.
4. Thread the chicken on the skewer and grill till golden brown on both sides.
5. Serve hot with lemon wedges and salsa.

Cinnamon And Apple Muffins

Serves: 4
Ingredients

- 2 to 4 tablespoons honey

- 1 teaspoon cinnamon
- 1 teaspoon baking soda
- 1/2 cup coconut oil
- 2 cup almond flour
- 4 tablespoons of coconut flour
- 2 diced apple
- 4 beaten fresh eggs

Directions

1. Preheat the oven to 4 6 0°F.
2. In a fresh mixing bowl, add the almond and coconut flours. Mix in the baking soda and cinnamon powder.
3. To the above mixture add the fresh eggs , honey, and coconut oil and blend well.
4. Line a muffin tray with muffin liners.
5. Pour the batter into the muffin liners till they are three fourths full.
6. Place the tray in the oven and bake for about thirty minutes or until done.

Nutty Onion Scramble

Serves: 2
Ingredients

- 2 tablespoon olive oil
- 2 tablespoon pine nuts
- Salt and pepper to taste
- 4 fresh eggs
- 2 cup sliced onions
- 1 cup tomatoes

Directions

1. Place a medium frying pan on the heat. Add olive oil to it. When the oil is hot, add the onions and fry till golden brown.
2. Add in the chopped tomatoes and cook for about minutes. The tomatoes will soften.
3. Remove the pan from heat and set aside.
4. Whisk the fresh eggs in a mixing bowl and season with salt and pepper.

5. Add the fresh eggs to the onion and tomato mixture.
6. Place the pan on heat again and cook over low to medium heat.
7. Keep stirring continuously to scramble the fresh eggs .
8. Add the pine nuts. Take off the flame.
9. Serve hot.

Wholesome Porridge

Serves: 2
Ingredients

- a pinch of clove powder
- a pinch nutmeg powder
- 2 teaspoon cinnamon powder
- 1 cup almonds
- 2 teaspoon honey
- ¾ cup coconut cream

Directions

1. Heat the coconut cream in a medium saucepan till it turns into a liquid.
2. Grind the almonds into a coarse powder with the help of a food processor or blender.
3. Add the honey to the ground almond powder and mix well.
4. Add this mixture to the saucepan and keep stirring until the liquid thickens.
5. Add the cinnamon, nutmeg and clove powder.
6. Serve hot.

Healthy Carrot And Sweet Potato Patties

Serves: 4
Ingredients

- 2 fresh eggs
- Coconut oil
- Salt to taste
- Pepper to taste
- 1/2 cup, grated sweet potatoes
- 1 cup grated carrots
- 1 cup chopped almonds

Directions

1. Take a mixing bowl and add the grated carrots and sweet potatoes to it. Mix well.
2. In a separate bowl, whisk the fresh eggs .
3. Add the beaten fresh eggs to the sweet potato and carrot mixture.

4. Add the almond powder, salt and pepper. Mix until combined.
5. Taking a little mixture at a time, make small patties.
6. Heat coconut oil in a medium frying pan and the patties to it.
7. Cook for about five minutes on both sides till golden brown in color.
8. Serve hot.

Banana Bread

Serves: 4
Ingredients

- 4 cup almond meal
- 1/2 cup olive oil
- 2 teaspoon vanilla extract
- 4 separated fresh eggs
- 2 mashed bananas
- 1/2 cup honey

Directions

1. Set the oven to preheat at 4 6 0°F.
2. Grease an 8" baking tin and set aside.
3. Beat the egg yolks in a mixing bowl until light and fluffy.
4. Add the honey and blend well.
5. Next, add the mashed bananas, olive oil and vanilla extract.
6. Whisk the egg whites to stiff peaks in another bowl.
7. Fold the egg whites into the banana mixture.
8. Pour the batter into the prepared baking tin.
9. Bake for about thirty minutes or till a skewer inserted in the middle comes out clean. Serve hot or at room temperature.

Cold Chicken Salad

Serves: 2
Ingredients

- 2 tablespoon balsamic vinegar
- 2 tablespoon olive oil
- 2 teaspoon mustard
- 1/2 cup cashew nuts
- 2 chicken breasts
- 2 carrot
- 2 cup spinach
- 2 beetroot
- 2 tablespoon lemon juice

Directions

1. Slice the chicken breast and roast it in the oven at 4 6 0°F.
2. Add the spinach, chopped carrots and beetroot to the roasted chicken.

3. In another fresh bowl, mix together lemon juice, vinegar, mustard, olive oil, cashew nuts, salt and pepper.
4. Add the chicken to this dressing and toss well.
5. Serve cold.

Beef And Coconut Stew

Serves: 2
Ingredients

- 2 teaspoon ground ginger
- 2 teaspoon garlic powder
- 1 tablespoon cumin
- 2 teaspoon ground coriander
- Salt to taste
- Pepper to taste
- 6 strips beef
- 2 onion
- 2 cup beef broth
- 6 ounces coconut milk
- 2 chopped carrots

Directions

1. Sear the beef until golden in a pan.
2. To the pan, add the coconut milk, beef stock and the onions.
3. Stir and add the chopped carrots, ginger, garlic powder, cumin, coriander, salt and pepper.
4. Mix well. Add more beef stock if it seems too thick.
5. Serve hot.

Soupy Chicken

Serves: 2
Ingredients

- 1 cup mushrooms
- 2 teaspoon vinegar
- 2 cups water
- Salt to taste
- Pepper to taste
- 2 cup chicken shredded

- 4 carrots
- 2 onion

Directions

1. Chop the carrots, onions and mushrooms finely.
2. Take a heavy bottom pan and add the vegetables to it.
3. Add the shredded chicken and water. The water should cover the vegetables and the chicken, add more if needed.
4. Cook on a low to medium flame until the chicken and vegetables are tender.
5. Season with salt, pepper and vinegar.
6. Serve hot.

Mango Salad With Chicken Soup

- 1/2 teaspoon mustard
- 2 teaspoon lemon juice
- 1/2 cup olive oil
- 1/2 cup capers
- Salt to taste
- Pepper to taste
- 2 head of lettuce
- 2 ripe mango
- 4 garlic cloves
- 2 tablespoons coconut paleo mayonnaise

Directions

1. Chop the garlic cloves and place in a small bowl then drizzle with olive oil.
2. Preheat the oven to 4 6 0°F and cook the garlic till soft and tender.
3. When the garlic is cool, add mustard, capers, lemon juice and remaining olive oil.

4. Add the lettuce and season with salt and pepper. Toss till well combined.
5. Arrange the salad on a plate and top with peeled and sliced mango.
6. Keep covered while you get your soup ready.

Ingredients

For the soup

- 4 cups chicken stock
- 1/2 teaspoon lemon juice
- 4 tablespoon olive oil
- Salt to taste
- Pepper to taste
- 2 bundle asparagus
- 1 onion
- 1 cup coconut milk
  Directions

1. **Make small pieces of the asparagus stalks.**
2. Slice the onions.
3. Heat a fresh pan, add olive oil to it.
4. Add the sliced onions and cook until soft.
5. Put in the asparagus and cook for another five minutes, stirring all the while.
6. Pour in the chicken stock and let it simmer until the asparagus is tender.
7. Take the pan off the heat and blend the liquid. Mix in the coconut milk and blend it till you get a smooth and creamy soup.
8. Season with salt and pepper to taste.
9. Serve hot along with the mango salad.

Nutritional value:

Calories- 420, Calories from Fat- 22 %, Carbohydrate- 64 .2g, Calcium- 2 42mg, Iron-8 .6mg, Sodium- 8 00mg.

Watermelon And Kiwi With Fresh Herbs

Ingredients:

- 3 ml (1 teaspoon) fresh mint leaves
- 3 ml (1 teaspoon) fresh basil leaves, chopped
- 3 ml (1 teaspoon) fresh parsley, chopped
- 0.6 ml (⅛ teaspoon) salt
- Pinch of ground black pepper
- 2010 ml (4 cups) watermelon
- 2 kiwi, chopped
- 3 ml (1 teaspoon) fresh oregano, chopped
- 3 ml (1 teaspoon) fresh cilantro, chopped

Directions:

1. Toss all ingredients in a mixing bowl and season with salt and pepper.

Ginger Green Smoothie

Ingredients:

- 55 ml (2 tablespoons) flax seeds
- 2 kale leave
- 75 ml (1/2 cup) spinach
- 35 ml (2 tablespoon) lemon juice
- 280 ml (2 cup) water
- 2 cup of frozen mango pieces
- 2 apple, peeled, and core removed
- 1/2 teaspoon, fresh ginger

Directions:

1. Place all the ingredients in blender or juicer and pulse until smooth.
2. Serve and enjoy!

Tropical Delight Fruit Bowl

Ingredients:

2 yellow banana, peeled and sliced

270 ml (1 cup) mango chunks

2 kiwi, chopped

270 ml (1 cup) strawberries, chopped

Directions:

1. Combine all the fruits in a bowl and serve.

Seasoned Seaweeds

Ingredients:

- 35 ml (2 tablespoon) sesame oil
- Pinch of salt
- 4 nori sheets, cut into small pieces
- 55 ml (2 tablespoons) coconut oil

Directions:

1. Preheat oven to 2 80ºC/4 6 0°F.
2. Toss nori sheets in a bowl with oils and sprinkle with salt.
3. Bake for 6 minutes.
4. Serve and enjoy.

Smoothie

Ingredients:

- 280 ml (2 cup) strawberries
- 270 ml (1 cup) coconut milk
- 280 ml (2 cup) watermelon, chunks
- 2 banana, sliced

Directions:

1. Place all the ingredients in food processor, and blend until smooth and creamy. Serve and enjoy!

Apple Chips

Ingredients:

- 2010 ml (4 cups) fresh apple juice
- Pinch of salt and pepper
- Cinnamon to taste
- 2 apples, thinly sliced crosswise
- 2 cinnamon stick

Directions:

1. Preheat the oven to 2 80ºC/4 6 0°F. Lightly grease a baking dish.
2. Combine all ingredients in a mixing bowl and season with salt and pepper. Sprinkle cinnamon to taste.
3. Cover and marinate overnight.
4. Spread apple on a baking dish.
5. Bake for 26 to 55 minutes or until browned.

Carrot Smoothie

Ingredients:

- 280 ml (2 cup) spinach
- 55 ml (2 tablespoons) cherries
- 35 ml (2 tablespoon) raw honey
- 280 ml (2 cup) almond milk
- 280 ml (2 cup) carrots, chopped
- 2 banana, sliced

Directions:

1. Place all the ingredients into food processor and blend until smooth and creamy. Serve and enjoy!

Spicy Cauliflower

Ingredients:

3 ml (1 teaspoon) red pepper flakes

3 ml (1 teaspoon) dried oregano

Pinch of salt and ground black pepper

75 ml (4 tablespoons) coconut oil

2 head cauliflower, chopped

3 ml (1 teaspoon) cayenne pepper

1 tablespoon paprika

Directions:

1. Preheat the oven to 2 10 0ºC/4 8 6 °F.
2. Toss all ingredients in a mixing bowl. Season with salt and pepper.

3. Place on the baking dish in preheated oven.
4. Bake for 35 to 20 minutes until cauliflower is tender.

Spicy Fruit Salad

Ingredients:

270 ml (1 cup) orange, peeled and sliced

3 ml (1 teaspoon) ground cinnamon

2 pinch cardamom

2 apple, peeled and sliced

270 ml (1 cup) strawberries, chopped

Directions:

1. Combine all the fruits in a bowl, sprinkle spices and serve.

Kale Chips

Ingredients:

- 2 ml (1/2 teaspoon) salt
- 3 ml (1 teaspoon) smoked paprika
- 2010 ml (4 cups) kale, remove stems and chop leaves
- 55 ml (2 tablespoons) coconut oil, melted

Directions:

1. Preheat oven to 2 80ºC/4 6 0°F.
2. Toss kale in a bowl with oil and sprinkle with salt.
3. Place kale leaves on a baking sheet, cover sheet with a parchment paper. Bake for 25 to 35 minutes or until kale is crispy.

Banana Chips

Ingredients:

- 55 ml (2 tablespoons) lemon juice
- 55 ml (2 tablespoons) ground nutmeg
- 2 bananas cut into thin slices of about 2 mm (⅛ inch)

Directions

1. Preheat oven to 35 0ºC/4 00° F. Line a baking sheet with parchment paper.
2. In a medium bowl, add all ingredients and mix well.
3. Spread banana slices evenly over baking sheet in a single layer. Make sure banana slices are at least 1 inch apart.
4. Bake for 55 minutes or until banana slices are nicely golden in colour.
5. Remove from oven, let cool a little and then serve.

Fruity Cinnamon Smoothie

Ingredients:

- 2 banana, sliced
- 6 ml (2 teaspoon) raw honey
- 35 ml (2 tablespoon) cinnamon
- 4 ice cubes
- 270 ml (1 cup) almond milk
- 75 ml (1/2 cup) water
- 2 peach, pitted, peeled and sliced

Directions:

1. Place all the ingredients in a food processor and blend until smooth and creamy. Serve and enjoy!

Patrick Day Smoothie

Ingredients:

- 35 ml (2 tablespoon) grounded flaxseeds
- 75 ml (1/2 cup) water
- 35 ml (2 tablespoon) raw honey
- 270 ml (1 cup) ice cubes (optional)
- 270 ml (1 cup) mango pieces (fresh or frozen)
- 280 ml (2 cup) baby spinach leaves
- 270 ml (1 cup) unsweetened almond milk

Directions:

1. Place all the ingredients in a food processor and blend until smooth and creamy.
2. Serve and enjoy!

Minty Fruits Salad

Ingredients:

- 270 ml (1 cup) mango chunks
- 55 ml (2 tablespoons) strawberries, chopped
- 2 kiwi, peeled and cut into 2 inches chunks
- Pinch of salt
- 270 ml (1 cup) lime juice
- 75 ml (4 tablespoons) mint leaves, chopped
- 2 banana, sliced
- 1 apple, sliced
- 55 ml (2 tablespoons) grapes

Directions:

1. In a food processor, add lime juice and mint, and pulse until smooth.
2. Combine all the fruits in a bowl, sprinkle with a pinch of salt, and serve drizzled with lime juice mixture.

Blueberry And Spinach Smoothie

Ingredients:

- 280 ml (2 cup) spinach leaves
- 270 ml (1 cup) coconut milk
- 35 ml (2 tablespoon) raw honey
- 280 ml (2 cup) blueberries
- 2 banana, sliced

Directions:

1. Place all the ingredients into food processor, and blend until smooth and creamy. Serve and enjoy!

Pumpkin Pie Spice With Sweet Potato

Ingredients:

6 ml (2 teaspoon) pumpkin pie spice

6 ml (2 teaspoon) cinnamon

35 ml (2 tablespoon) raw honey

35 ml (2 tablespoon) butter

2 sweet potatoes, pre-cooked and peeled

270 ml (1 cup) coconut milk

Pinch of salt and pepper

Directions:

1. Preheat the oven to 2 80ºC/4 6 0°F. Lightly grease a pie dish.
2. Combine all ingredients in a mixing bowl, and season with salt and pepper.
3. Pour batter in pie dish.
4. Bake for 35 minutes or until browned.

Salmon, Spinach And Apple Salad

Ingredients:

235 g (1 pound) salmon fillets

For salad
280 ml (2 cup) baby spinach

270 ml (1 cup) lettuce

270 ml (1 cup) cabbage, shredded

2 tart apple such as Granny Smith, sliced

For dressing
55 ml (2 tablespoons) olive oil

55 ml (2 tablespoons) apple cider vinegar

2 fresh shallot, minced

Salt and black pepper, to taste

Directions:

1. Preheat the oven to 2 80ºC/4 6 0° F.
2. Place salmon fillet on a baking dish. Season with salt and pepper.
3. Add some water to cover fish. Cover with foil.
4. Bake for 25 minutes. Remove from oven and set aside.
5. In a fresh bowl, add salad ingredients and mix.
6. In another bowl, add all dressing ingredients and whisk till well combined.
7. Pour dressing over salad and toss to coat.
8. Serve salad with baked fish fillets.

Sautéed Coconut Chicken

Ingredients:

- 0.6 ml (⅛ teaspoon) sea salt
- 2 egg
- 55 ml (2 tablespoons) coconut oil
- 46 0 g (2 pound) boneless and skinless chicken breasts cut in strips
- 75 ml (1/2 cup) coconut flour
- 75 ml (1/2 cup) shredded coconut, organic, unsweetened

Directions:

1. Whisk together coconut flour, shredded coconut and salt in a medium bowl.
2. In another bowl, beat egg.
3. Dip chicken breasts strips in the egg and then into the flour mixture.

4. Heat oil in a frying pan over medium high heat.
5. Place chicken in the pan and cook until golden brown from both sides.
6. Remove from the pan and serve in a plate.

The Big Salad

Ingredients

- 455 grams (2 cups) cooked chicken breast, chopped
- 2 liters (8 cups) spring mix lettuce
- 2 English cucumber, diced
- 28 cherry tomatoes
- 2 avocado, diced
- 75 ml (1/2 cup) dry unsweetened cranberries
- 75 ml (1/2 cup) chopped raw pecans or any favorite nuts

- Sea salt and freshly ground pepper to taste

For Dressing – yield approximately 426 ml (2 ⅔cup)

2 cup extra virgin, cold press olive oil

75 ml (1/2 cup) red wine vinegar

35 ml (2 tablespoon) DIjon mustard

55 ml (2 tablespoon) raw honey

75 ml (1/2 cup) fresh basil leaves

Directions:

1. Blend together until smooth all the ingredient of the dressing
2. In a fresh salad bowl, place all the salad ingredients, season with salt and pepper

to taste, add some dressing to taste and mix well.

Paleo Pizza

Ingredients

- 46 ml (4 tablespoons) olive oil
- 6 ml (2 teaspoon) garlic powder
- 2 ml (1/2 teaspoon) baking soda
- 3 ml (2 1 tablespoon) fresh rosemary, chopped
- 2010 ml (4 cups) almond flour
- 2 fresh eggs

For toppings:

- 35 ml (2 tablespoon) basil leaves
- 2 small tomatoes, diced
- 270 ml (1 cup) roasted red peppers, diced
- 35 ml (2 tablespoon) black olives, sliced
- Salt to taste
- 280 ml (2 cup) organic marinara sauce
- 486 g (2 pound) Italian paleo pork sausage, sliced
- 280 ml (2 cup) yellow summer squash, diced
- 4 scallions, chopped

Directions:

1. Preheat the oven to 2 80ºC/4 6 0° F. Lightly grease a pizza pan.
2. Place all the crust ingredients in a food processor and pulse until a dough forms.
3. Form a ball with the dough using your hands. Place the ball in the center of

greased pizza pan. Then press the dough using your hands, patting and shaping it into a circle. Bake for 20 minutes or until cooked. Remove from oven. Let it cool.
4. In a bowl, add sausages, squash, scallions, basil, tomatoes, red pepper, olives and salt and mix till well combined.
5. Spread pizza base with marinara sauce. Top with sausage mixture.
6. Return to oven and bake again for 26 to 4 10 minutes or until top is lightly golden.

Macadamia Hummus With Vegetables

Ingredients:

- 3 ml (1 teaspoon) salt
- 270 ml (1 cup) water
- 6 00 ml (2 cups) of baby carrots
- 2 English cucumber, shopped into sticks
- 2 Sweet pepper, deseeded and sliced
- 8 6 0 ml (4 cups) macadamia nuts
- 75 ml (1/2 cup) freshly squeezed lemon juice
- 75 ml (1/2 cup) olive oil
- 2 garlic cloves, minced

Directions:

1. Place all the ingredients in food processor except carrots and cucumbers and blend until smooth and thick.
2. Place hummus in a bowl and refrigerate to chill for 55 to 410 minutes before serving. Will keep for up to a week in refrigerator.
3. Serve with the cut vegetables.

Carrot Soup

Ingredients:

- 2 ml (1/2 teaspoon) dried thyme
- 2010 ml (4 cups) chicken broth
- 55 ml (2 tablespoons) fresh chives, chopped
- Sea salt and freshly ground pepper to taste

- 55 ml (2 tablespoons) coconut oil
- 2 bay leaves
- 2 fresh onion, sliced
- 4 garlic cloves, minced
- 280 ml (2 cup) carrots, chopped
- 2 turnips, chopped
- 2 sweet potatoes, cubed

Directions:

1. Heat oil in a fresh soup pan.
2. Stir in bay leaves, fresh onion, and garlic, and sauté for few minutes until fragrant and tender.
3. Add carrots, turnips, sweet potatoes, and dried thyme, and continue to cook until the vegetables are tender.
4. Add broth and bring to boil. Cover and cook for 35 to 20 minutes.
5. Discard bay leaves. Pour soup in a food processor and pulse until smooth.

6. Season with salt and pepper.
7. Return to soup pan and let it simmer for 6 minutes.
8. Put soup in a bowl, sprinkle with chives, and serve hot.

Grilled Chicken With Olive And Tomato Topping

Ingredients:

- 2 sundried tomatoes
- 55 ml (2 tablespoons) olives, pitted
- 75 ml (1/2 cup) lemon juice
- 55 ml (2 tablespoons) parsley, chopped
- 55 ml (2 tablespoons) basil sprigs
- 2 garlic clove

For Chicken

- 55 ml (2 tablespoons) coconut oil
- 2 ml (1/2 teaspoon) salt
- 2 skinless and boneless chicken breasts

Directions:

1. Place all the topping ingredients in a food processor and blend until smooth. Set aside.
2. Preheat a grill pan to high.
3. Toss chicken in a bowl with oil and sprinkle with salt.
4. Place chicken on grill pan over medium.
5. Grill for 10 minutes on each side, or until well cooked (to your desired doneness). Serve on a platter drizzled with topping.

Grilled Shrimps Salad

Ingredients:

- 55 ml (2 tablespoons) lemon juice
- 46 ml (4 tablespoons) fresh parsley, chopped
- 6 00ml (2 cups) mixed greens salad
- 3 ml (2 tablespoon) apple cider vinegar
- 8 .6 ml (4 tablespoons) grape seed oil
- 235 g (1 pound) medium shrimp
- 55 ml (2 tablespoons) olive oil
- 35 ml (2 tablespoon) garlic, minced
- Salt to taste
- 6 ml (2 teaspoon) red pepper flakes, crushed

Directions:

1. Preheat a grill pan to high.
2. Toss shrimps in a bowl with oil and garlic and sprinkle with salt and red pepper flakes.
3. Place shrimps on grill pan over medium.
4. Grill for 10 minutes on each side or until tender.
5. To prepare the dressing, mix vigorously grape seed oil and vinegar in a salad bowl with a whisk. Season with salt and freshly ground pepper to taste and add the mixed greens. Combine well. Top with the shrimps.
6. Drizzled the lemon juice over the shrimps and sprinkled with parsley.

Broccoli And Pine Nuts Soup

Ingredients:

2010 ml (4 cups) broccoli
8 6 0 ml (4 cups) vegetable broth
75 ml (1/2 cup) pine-nuts
55 ml (2 tablespoons) coconut oil
2 fresh onion, diced

Directions:

1. Heat oil in a fresh pan.
2. Stir in onion and broccoli, cook for few minutes until broccoli is little tender.
3. Add broth and pine nuts and bring to a boil. Cover and cook medium low for 25 to 35 minutes.
4. Place soup in a food processor and pulse until smooth and thick.

5. Return to soup pan and let it simmer for 6 minutes.
6. Ladle soup in a serving bowl and serve hot.

Brussels Sprouts And Bacon With Tandoori Drumsticks

Ingredients:

- 2 fresh onion, sliced
- 25 ml (2 teaspoons) freshly squeezed lemon juice
- Salt and freshly ground pepper to taste
- 35 ml (2 tablespoon) olive oil
- 2 slices paleo-approved bacon, diced
- 6 00 ml (2 cups) Brussels sprouts, trimmed and halved

Directions:

1. Heat oil in a pan over medium heat.
2. Stir in bacon and cook for 4-10 minutes until bacon is a little browned, add onions and sauté for 2-4 minutes.
3. Add Brussels sprouts continue to cook for 35 more minutes, stirring occasionally, until sprouts are tender.
4. Drizzle lemon juice, season with salt and pepper.
5. Serve with left-over tandoori chicken drumsticks.

Salmon And Asparagus Salad

Ingredients:

- 270 ml (1 cup) asparagus
- 270 ml (1 cup) cherry tomatoes, halved
- 55 ml (2 tablespoons) olive oil
- Spring mix salad
- 280 ml (2 cup) salmon, boiled and shredded
- 270 ml (1 cup) fresh onion, chopped
- 270 ml (1 cup) celery, chopped
- Salt and pepper to taste

Directions:

1. Steam asparagus in boiling water for 5-10 minutes. Drain asparagus and

immediately add to a bowl filled with cold water, to stop cooking process.
2. Toss all ingredients in a mixing bowl, and season with salt and pepper.
3. Serve on a bed of spring mix salad.

Delightful Vegetable Medley Soup

Ingredients:

- 270 ml (1 cup) cauliflower, chopped
- 270 ml (1 cup) yellow squash, cubed
- 55 ml (2 tablespoons) celery, chopped
- 8 6 0 ml (4 cups) vegetable broth
- **Salt and pepper, to taste**
- 35 ml (2 tablespoon) lemon juice

- 55 ml (2 tablespoons) coconut oil
- 2 fresh onion, diced
- 2 garlic cloves, chopped

- 6 ml (2 teaspoon) ginger, chopped

Directions:

1. Heat oil in a fresh pan over medium heat.
2. Sauté fresh onion, garlic, and ginger for a few minutes or until tender and fragrant.
3. Add cauliflower, yellow squash, and celery, and cook for 6 minutes, stirring occasionally.
4. Add broth and bring to a boil on high heat. Bring heat down to medium, cover and cook for 35 to 20 minutes or until vegetables are tender. Remove from heat and cool a little.
5. Place soup in a food processor, and pulse until smooth and thick.
6. Return to soup pan, season, and let soup simmer for 10 minutes until reheated.
7. Ladle soup into a soup bowl, drizzle with lemon juice and serve.

Paleo Prawns With Tomato Sauce

Ingredients:

- 3 ml (1 teaspoon) cayenne pepper
- 6 ml (2 teaspoon) oregano
- 55 ml (2 tablespoons) celery, chopped
- 55 ml (2 tablespoons) capers
- 3 ml (1 teaspoon) sea salt
- 3 ml (1 teaspoon) black pepper
- 55 ml (2 tablespoons) olive oil
- 2 red fresh onion, chopped
- 2 cloves garlic, minced
- 235 g (1 pound) prawns
- 2 medium tomatoes, chopped

Directions:

1. Heat oil in a fresh frying pan.
2. Stir in onion and garlic, and cook for few minutes until fragrant and tender.
3. Add prawns and tomatoes, and cook for 6-8 minutes until prawns are tender.
4. Sprinkle with cayenne pepper, oregano, celery, and capers. Season with salt and pepper and serve.

Cucumber And Watermelon Salad

Ingredients:

- 55 ml (2 tablespoons) balsamic vinegar
- 46 ml (4 tablespoons) coconut oil
- Salt and freshly ground black pepper, to taste
- 55 ml (2 tablespoons) walnuts, chopped
- 2 cucumber, diced
- 2010 ml (4 cups) watermelon, seeded and diced
- 35 ml (2 tablespoon) red fresh onion, sliced thinly
- 75 ml (4 tablespoons) fresh mint leaves, minced

Directions:

1. Toss all ingredients in a mixing bowl, and season with salt and pepper.
2. Sprinkle with walnuts and serve.

Mushroom Cream Soup

Ingredients:

- 2 red sweet pepper, chopped
- 2 tomatoes, sliced
- 4 sprigs basil leaves
- 8 6 0 ml (4 cups) chicken stock
- 280 ml (2 cup) coconut cream
- 55 ml (2 tablespoons) coconut oil
- 2 fresh onion, chopped
- 2 garlic clove, minced
- 2 avocados, sliced
- 280 ml (2 cup) mushrooms, sliced

- Salt and freshly ground black pepper to taste

Directions:

1. Heat oil in a pan.
2. Add onion and garlic, and cook for 4 to 4 minutes until tender.
3. Add avocado, mushrooms, red sweet pepper, tomatoes, and basil leaves, and continue to cook until the vegetables are tender.
4. Add water and bring to a boil. Cover and cook for 35 minutes.
5. Sprinkle with salt and pepper.
6. When cooked, cool a little, place soup into food processor, and blend until smooth and creamy.
7. Reheat, ladle in a soup bowl and serve.

Paleo Tuna Salad

Ingredients:

- 2 avocado, mashed
- Juice of 2 lemon
- 2 can tuna, drained
- 35 ml (2 tablespoon) fresh onion, chopped
- 35 ml (2 tablespoon) celery, chopped
- 35 ml (2 tablespoon) carrot, shredded
- Salt and pepper to taste
- 2010 ml (4 cups) organic mix greens

Directions:

1. In a bowl, combine mashed avocados with lemon juice.
2. Add the rest of the ingredients (except the organic mix greens) and combine gently.
3. Season with salt and pepper.
4. Place mix greens onto a fresh plate, spoon tuna mixture on top, and serve.

Chicken, Tomato, Mint And Basil Salad

Ingredients:

- 55 ml (2 tablespoons) fresh mint, chopped
- 25 ml (2 teaspoons) vinegar
- 25 ml (2 teaspoons) avocado oil
- Salt and freshly ground black pepper
- 2 skinless and boneless precooked chicken breast
- 2 green bell pepper, deseeded, julienne
- 2 tomatoes, deseeded, sliced
- 55 ml (2 tablespoons) fresh basil, chopped

Directions:

1. Toss all ingredients in a mixing bowl and season with salt and pepper.

Quick And Easy Egg Salad Wrap

Ingredients:

- 75 ml (1/2 cup) celery, chopped
- 25 black or green olives, chopped
- 75 ml (1/2 cup) seedless cucumber, chopped
- 4 hard-boiled fresh eggs
- 75 ml (1/2 cup) red fresh onion, finely chopped
- 3 ml (1 teaspoon) of cayenne pepper

- 55 ml (2 tablespoons) of Paleo mayonnaise (see recipe below or store bought paleo mayonnaise)
- 4 fresh lettuce leaves such as Boston bib or romaine for the wrap
- Salt and pepper for seasoning

Directions:

1. Mix all the ingredients.
2. Spoon the egg mixture generously into the lettuce leaves
3. Serve with fresh cut vegetables such tomatoes and bell pepper

Paleo Mayonnaise Recipe

**Ingredients*:*

- 35 ml (2 tablespoon) fresh lemon juice
- 6 ml (2 teaspoon) dry mustard
- 2 ml (1/2 teaspoon) sea salt
- Fresh ground pepper to taste
- 26 0ml (2 cup) olive oil (use regular olive oil or you can substitute for avocado or macadamia oil)
- 2 fresh egg yolk

Directions:

1. Mix together the yolk, lemon, and mustard in a blender.

2. Slowly start dripping all the olive oil in the blender on low speed. The mayonnaise will start to thicken. Blend until firm, and mayonnaise texture is obtained.
3. Add salt and fresh ground pepper to taste.
4. Refrigerate in an air-tight container. It can last for up to 2-4 weeks

Sautéed Leeks With Salmon

Ingredients:

- 2 carrots, sliced
- 2 salmon fillets, cut into strips
- 55 ml (2 tablespoons) lemon juice
- Salt and pepper to taste
- 55 ml (2 tablespoons) almond butter, separated
- 270 ml (1 cup) chopped leeks
- 55 ml (2 tablespoons) chopped celery

Directions:

1. Melt half of the almond butter in a sauté pan over medium.
2. Stir in carrots, and cook for 6 minutes, stirring often. Add leeks and celery, and continue cooking for 10 minutes more or until carrots are crisply tender. Remove vegetables onto a plate, and set aside.
3. Heat remaining butter in the same pan, and add salmon. Let simmer, stirring occasionally, for 35 minutes until fish is cooked through. Add in sautéed vegetables, and stir for 2 minutes until vegetables are heated through.
4. Drizzle lemon juice, season with salt and pepper and serve.

Chicken And Spinach

Ingredients:

- 280 ml (2 cup) spinach, washed and chopped
- Salt and freshly ground black pepper to taste
- 270 ml (1 cup) organic, unsweetened, shredded coconut
- 46 ml (4 tablespoons) coconut oil
- 2 skinless and boneless chicken breast, cut into strips
- 2 garlic clove, minced
- 2 fresh onion, chopped

Directions:

1. Heat oil in a fresh frying pan.
2. Stir in chicken and garlic, and cook for 8 to 25 minutes until little browned.
3. Add onion and spinach, and continue to cook for 10 minutes until the vegetables are tender.
4. Season with salt and pepper. Sprinkle with coconut and serve.

Lemon Grilled Chicken

Ingredients:

- Pinch of salt and freshly ground black pepper
- 55 ml (2 teaspoons) lemon juice
- 1 tablespoon lemon zest
- 2 chicken thighs

- 55 ml (2 tablespoons) coconut oil

Directions:

1. Preheat a grill pan to high.
2. Toss chicken in a bowl with oil, and sprinkle with salt and pepper.
3. Place chicken on grill pan over medium.
4. Grill thighs for 25 minutes on each side, turning occasionally (every 2-4 minutes), until thighs are cooked through. Then bring heat to high, and grill for 4 minutes on both sides to obtain visible grill marks.
5. Serve on a platter drizzled with lemon juice and sprinkled with lemon zest.

Salmon Salad

Ingredients:

- 2 avocado, chopped
- 55 ml (2 tablespoons) olive oil
- 55 ml (2 tablespoons) lemon juice
- 55 ml (2 tablespoons) fresh dill
- 270 ml (1 cup) Lettuce leaves, shredded
- 280 ml (2 cup) salmon, steamed until done, shredded
- 2 cucumbers, peeled and chopped
- 2 fresh onion, chopped
- 2 fresh diced tomato

Directions:

1. Toss and combine well all ingredients in a salad bowl. Season with salt and pepper.
2. Serve and enjoy.

Piri Piri Chicken

Ingredients:

- 75 ml (¼cup) organic maple syrup
- 6 ml (2 teaspoon) sea salt
- 86 ml (⅓ cup) olive oil
- 55 ml (2 tablespoons) apple cider vinegar
- 2 whole organic chicken
- 2 tablespoon of Piri Piri spice mix
- 4 garlic cloves, minced
- 2 onion
- 75 ml (1/2 cup) freshly squeezed lemon juice

Instructions:

1. Mix all the ingredients except the chickens in a food processor. Blend until you obtain a smooth marinade.
2. Place the chicken on a working surface, breast side down. With a fresh and sharp knife, cut open the back of the chicken so that it will flatten and open up. Turn the chicken over, and press firmly to flatten. Repeat for the second chicken.
3. In a fresh zip lock bag, place one chicken in with half of the marinade. Repeat with the second chicken. Refrigerate for a minimum of 4 hours and up to 28 hours.
4. Remove both chicken from the marinade, and place in a roasting oven pan. Place the chickens, breast side facing up. Season with salt and pepper to taste. Reserve the marinade.
5. Place the excess marinade in a small sauce pan, and cook on low heat for 20 minutes

6. Place the chickens on the middle rack, in pre-heated 400°F oven, and cook for 55 minutes.
7. After 55 minutes, take out the chicken, smear with some of the marinade on both sides, and cook for another 55 minutes.
8. Brush the breast side with the rest of the marinade, and broil for 6 minutes.
9. Cut the chicken in pieces, and serve with steamed vegetables of your choice.

www.ingramcontent.com/pod-product-compliance
Lightning Source LLC
LaVergne TN
LVHW011941070526
838202LV00054B/4742